CANCER
CAN
STRIKE
ANYONE..
ANYTIME..

You Deserve

Preface

You can really prevent cancer from occurring and if afflicted by cancer then you can greatly recover from it by following these procedures. If you are looking for optional treatment of cancer, then the alternative means can certainly aid you in coping with signs and symptoms caused by cancer and cancer treatments. This Books Bring to you all cancer cures available in modern medical science and would be of great help for patients and families fighting Cancer.

Table of Content

You can lessen your danger for cancer. You must not wait for diagnosis as you have to take measures for prevention. It is much uncomplicated to prevent cancer than to treat the disease. You can really prevent cancer from occurring and if afflicted by cancer then you can greatly recover from it by following these procedures. If you are looking for optional treatment of cancer, then the alternative means can certainly aid you in coping with signs and symptoms caused by cancer and cancer treatments. Common signs and symptoms such as anxiety, fatigue, nausea and vomiting, pain, difficulty sleeping, and stress may be lessened by alternative treatments. Common signs and symptoms such as anxiety, fatigue, nausea and vomiting, pain, difficulty sleeping, and stress may be lessened by alternative treatments.

Food Preparation

If you are having foodstuff then eat at least a raw food. Try to avoid frying, charbroiling, boil or steaming your foodstuff. Include cancer-fighting complete foods spices, supplements herbs like curcumin, resveratol and broccoli..

Genetically Engineered Foods

Avoid genetically engineered foods as they are usually treated with herbicides like Roundup (glyphosate) and are cryogenic in nature.

Carbohydrates and Sugar

Try to minimize or eradicate processed foods and grain related foods from your diet as far as possible. They speedily break down and force up your insulin intensity. It is quite evident that if you want to prevent cancer or if you are suffering from cancer then you must try to ignore all sorts of sugars particularly fructose which feeds cancer cells and aids in growth of cancer. You must be quite certain that total fructose intake must be 25 grams per day including fruits.

Animal-Based Omega-3 fats- One can balance the ratio of omega-3 to omega-6 fats by taking a superior quality krill oil and minimizing the use of processed vegetable oils.

Alternative Cure helps people with cancer

Alternative cancer treatments might not play an unswerving role in healing your cancer, but they might help you to deal with signs and indications caused by cancer plus cancer treatments. Widespread signs furthermore symptoms such as nervousness, exhaustion, nausea and queasiness, sting, complexity sleeping, and strain possibly will be lessened by different treatments.

You have got to labor intimately with your doctor in knowing the precise eq equilibrium between the customary drugs along with voluntary cancer therapies. You have to converse in detail with your physician about the approach that would be rather conducive in healing the ailment. Whilst complimentary cancer remedial like acupuncture might lessen the aching but they are not burly enough to reinstate cancer drugs from your physician. If cancer makes you feel as if you have petite control over your wellbeing, substitute cancer cure might present some emotion of control. However lots of alternative cancer handling is original and some might even be risky.

The treatments you get from your physician may aid ease numerous of the sign linked with cancer as well as its healing. Converses all of your choice with your doctor in addition to together you can decide which policy might be better for you and which are probably to have no profit. Work directly with your general practitioner to establish the right poise between conventional medicines and substitute cancer cure. Though matching and substitute cancer cure, such as acupuncture, possibly will lessen nausea or ache, they usually aren't powerful enough to reinstate cancer medication from your physician.

If you are feeling anxiety then think about trying kneading, reflection, hypnosis and repose process. If you are quite tired then attempt to work out, massage, repose techniques and yoga would be fine enough. Similarly there is a ache in your body then try acupuncture, rub down, music treatment, aromatherapy as well as hypnosis. If you have sleeping problem then do exercise, yoga and follow relaxation method. If having stress then go for aromatherapy, tai chi, m

There are unusual surgeries are functional in curing cancer Surgery has been employed to cure cancer for a number of years. Surgery also plays a major role in studying cancer and knowing out how far the cancer has spread.). Ongoing progress in surgical course lets surgeons to function on a growing number of cancer patients and include fine results.

They depict a doctor via a scalpel and other surgical device to cut into plus eliminate, restore, or reinstate parts of the body affected by ailment. The newer techniques, utilizing diverse kinds of tool, have spread the idea of what in fact surgery is. A number of the methods are given in detail.

Laser surgery

A laser

A laser is considered to be greatly focused and effective ray of light energy utilized for very clear surgical task. It can be employed in its place of a blade or else scalpel to slash through tissue. It could also be utilized to blaze and spoil (vaporize) some cancers associated to cervix, lung, skin, or else other organs.

There are few laser surgeries which involve a smaller amount of cutting and smash up than normal operation. For instance, with strand optics and particular scopes the it can be aimed at within a normal body opening with no large cut. The laser is next accurately aimed to obliterate the tumor."

Cryosurgery

Cryosurgery utilizes a liquid nitrogen squirt or a very freezing probe to ice up and kill irregular cells. This system is from time to time utilized to take care of pre-cancerous situation such as those having an effect on the skin, cervix plus penis. Cryosurgery could also be practiced to heal some cancers such as those present in the liver moreover prostate. A scan such as an ultrasound or CT examination might be practiced to direct the check out into the disease and look at the cells solidify. This restrictions damages close by strong tissue.

Electro surgery

A high-rate electrical current is being utilized o wipe out cells. This might be done for few cancers such as of skin in addition to mouth.

Radiofrequency Ablation

This is known as RFA, consisting of high-energy radio effect are sent throughout a needle to warm up and annihilate cancer cells. RFA possibly will be utilized to take care of cancer tumors found in the kidney, liver, lungs and other body parts.

Mohs Surgery rate

Mohs micrographic surgery is also known as microscopically *restricted surgery*. It is practiced to eliminate definite skin cancers by means of shaving off one extremely thin coating at a time. After each layer is detached, the doctor observes the tissue through a microscope to make sure for cancer unit. The doctor recur this until the entire cells in a deposit appears normal.

Mohs surgical procedure is employed when the degree of the cancer is not identified or if healthy tissue as likely needs to be protected, like when curing skin cancers about the eye. The procedure is done by a particularly skilled doctor when the skin treated is insensitive.

Chemosurgery is a previous name for surgery and refers to definite drugs that may be put on the tissue before it's removed. Mohs surgery does not use chemotherapy drugs.

Laparoscopic surgery

A laparoscope is a stretched out, thin, stretchy tube that is capable of putting during a small cut to come out within the body. It's now and then exercised to take portions of tissue to analyze for cancer. In current years, doctors have set up that by creating minute holes and with special long, thin tool, the laparoscope be able to be utilized without building a huge cut. This can assist in decreasing blood loss during operation and pain later. It can also cut down hospital stays and let people to cure quicker. This surgery is utilized commonly nowadays to get rid of gallbladders, mend hernias, and for lots of other processes.

Laparoscopic surgical treatment is exercised in cancer treatment, however not for the entire cancers. Doctors can carefully and efficiently use laparoscopic surgeries intended for few cancers of the liver, rectum prostate, and kidney, amid others. Uses on other sorts of cancer are yet being studied.

Thorascopic surgery

A thoracoscope is a lean cylinder with a tiny video camera on the end that could be put throughout a small slash into the chest following the lung is malformed. This lets the doctor to perceive in the chest. This sort of surgery unswerving to less wounding and has yet been used to eliminate portion of the lung that has affected by cancer. Studies have revealed that for early-stage lung cancer is the cause using this means are much the similar as eliminating element of the lung through a slash in the region of the chest.

Robotic Surgery

Robotic surgery is a type of laparoscopic surgery where the physician sits at manages board and uses exact mechanical arms to administer the range and other particular tool. The advantages of this category of operation are frequently the identical as laparoscopic as well as thoracoscopic surgery: it is capable to aid in dipping blood loss during surgical procedure and ache afterward. It can in addition limit hospital stays and let people to cure sooner.

Robotic surgery is from time to time used to take care of cancers of the prostate, uterus as well as colon,, and it is employed in working on other parts is also being considered. It's not so far clear if mechanical surgery leads to improved long-term results as compared to operations where the general practitioner holds the device directly.

Other kinds of surgery

Doctors are all the time looking for novel ways to eradicate or wipe out cancer cells. Some of these processes smear the streak between what we frequently think of as operation and other forms of cure.

Researchers are trying a lot of new methods, like by means of high-intensity alert ultrasound, microwaves, plus even high-capacity magnets to endeavor to get free of ineffective tissue. These techniques are capable, but still mainly experimental.

. By using radiation basis from diverse angles, *stereotactic emission therapies bring* a large specific radiation amount to a minute tumor locale. The procedure is so precise that this is now and then described *stereotactic surgery*, although no cut is really made. In fact, the equipment used to carry this treatment has names similar to Gamma Knife and CyberKnife®, except no knife is implicated. The mind is the most widespread site that be able to be take care of using this method, but it's too used on a head, lung, spine, neck, and other tumors. Researchers are coming across for ways to employ it to care for other sort of cancer, too.

Chemotherapy

Chemotherapy is the utilization of tablets or drugs to heal cancer. The consideration of having chemotherapy scares lots of people. Although knowing the significance of chemotherapy is, how it functions, and what to suppose can often aid calm your qualms. It can also provide you a superior sense of managing over your cancer healing.

How to carry out chemo function?

The human body is equipped of trillions of common healthy cells. Cancer starts when something causes modification in a standard unit. This cancer unit after those develops out of control plus makes additional cancer cells. Each kind of cancer influences the body in diverse manner. If cancer is not taken care of, it can increase and affect the whole body.

Your doctor might propose chemo to heal your cancer.
From time to time the objective is to sluggish the enlargement of the cancer. Whereas other times the aim may be to lessen

symptoms or harms caused by increasing tumors so that you feel healthier. Chemo is repeatedly used to battle cancers that have extended to additional parts of the human body. Be sure to converse to your physician about the aim of your healing.

Chemo slays cancer cells. These medicines can affect common cells, also. But the majority of normal cells can patch up themselves.

Your cure will roughly use additional chemo medicine. This is known as *blend chemotherapy*. The drugs toil together to obliterate extra cancer cells.

How is chemo given?

Most chemo drugs are provided in one of these manners Now and then chemo is a capsule or liquid. You presently swallow it because your doctor recommends it. You can receive it at residence, but you have to be cautious to follow the instructions.

- Chemo be capable of be specified like a flu attempt. The shots might be specified in your doctor's workplace, a hospital, a health center, or at house.

- Most frequently, chemo pills are set into your blood all the way through a minuscule artificial pipe called a *catheter* that's lay in a seam. This is called chemo.
- Other sort of chemo can be lay right into the vertebrae, chest, or abdomen or stroke on the skin.

You might get chemo one time a day, one time a week, or still one time a month. It relies on the sort of cancer you contain and the pills you are receiving. Chemo is regularly offered with break amid treatment sequence. This break provides your body instance to restore strong new cells and aid you recover your potency. How time-consuming it would be, it depends on the kind of cancer, your healing goals, in addition to how your body react to the drugs.

Does chemo painful?

There might be a small ache while a spike is used but the tablets themselves must cause no soreness. If you do sense pain, ablaze, coolness, or something new when receiving your treatment, inform your physician or care for right away.

Can you take any other medicines while taking chemo?

Some other tablets can have an effect on your chemo. Be certain to inform your physician or nurse as regards all the drugs you intake. Don't overlook prescribed drugs in addition to the entire those you can get without a prescription. Also, inform them as regards vitamins, herbs, and whatever else you take for your fitness. Make and carry on a catalog of entire drugs you take. Keep this list up to date and allocate it with all your doctors.

Your doctor can tell you whether it's OK to take these drugs while you obtain chemo. Once you're healing start on, be certain to verify with your doctor prior to taking any new pills, and before you discontinue the pills you've been taking.

How one knows that chemo works?

The doctors plus nurses will observe the improvement in your fitness by doing bodily assessment, blood tests, as well as x-rays. Inquire your doctor to make clear any test fallout to you, and also prove improvement in your cure. You must keep in mind the side effects that you might encounter do not signify that the cure is — or is not — functioning.

Radiation healing uses high-energy element or waves to wipe out or injure cancer cells. It is considered as one of the largest common cure for cancer, moreover by itself or next to other type of cure.

How does radiation healing work?

The human body is created of trillions of usual, fit cells. Cancer begins when something alters a typical cell into a cancer unit. This cancer cell is capable of then expanding and creates more cancer cells unless a tumor is created. Tumors can continuously grow and cause harms. If the ailment is not cured, it can extend to other component and develop extra tumors.

Radiation is utilized to slay cancer cells. Extraordinary tools send high quantity of emission to the cancer unit or tumor. This creates more cancer cells. Energy can also influence standard cells close to the tumor. However standard cells can fix themselves and cancer unit cannot do so.

Sometimes emission is the just treatment desirable. Other time it is only part of a patient's ailment cure preparation.

Your doctor might advise radiation treatment for cancer. Sometimes emission can heal cancer. Sometimes the objective may be too unhurried the cancer's enlargements to assist you feel in good health. Be convinced to converse to your physician about the objective of your healing.

Radiation treatment is not similar to chemotherapy. Radiation treats the tumor. Chemo utilizes drugs to cure the whole body. Consequently chemo might be exploiting if a person has cancer in numerous parts. Radiation affects merely the part affected by cancer.

Taking care of yourself during rays

During emission therapy, you require to take particular heed of yourself. Your physician or nurse will offer you directives on how to perform this. However here are a few essential things that you ought to do:

- Get abundance of respite. You might feel extra tired than usual. This could last mean for 4 to 6 weeks following your healing ends and at times longer.
- Eat hale and hearty foods. Your general practitioner, nurse, or dietitian might toil with you to build sure you're consuming the accurate foods to acquire what your body wants. They might suggest modify to lessen side effects but your belly or gullet is in the region being taken care of.
- Take heed of the skin in the healing region. Dirt f free the skin every day with tepid water plus a gentle soap that your nurse utters is OK to employ. Don't utilize other goods on the healing area if your physician or nurse says to you its OK.
- Inform your doctor regarding all tablets you are taking. but you take some medicines, still aspirin, herbs, or else vitamins, allow your doctor be familiar with before you initiate vivacity.

Targeted treatment is a newer kind of cancer cure that make use of drugs or other material to more exactly recognize and bother cancer cells, typically as doing small harm to standard cells. Targeted healing is a rising part of numerous cancers healing schedule.

How does besieged cancer treatment work?

Most normal chemotherapy (chemo) drugs labor by slaying cells in the human body that produce and split rapidly. Cancer cells split swiftly, which is the main reason these drugs frequently toil against them. Other than chemo pills can also influence other unit in the body to divide rapidly, which can now and then lead to grave side effects. Beside, chemo drugs don't for all time work in opposition to cancer, or every now and then they discontinue working after a moment.

Targeted healing drugs work another way. These drugs aim definite division of cancer cells so as to make them dissimilar from other unit.

Cancer cells naturally have lots of transformation in their genes (DNA) to make them unlike from standard cells. These gene modification might be the reason for the cell to build extra of a definite protein, which in turn may formulate the cell raise and split too speedily. This sort of transformation is what formulate it a cancer cubicle.

But there are lots of unlike sort of cancer, and not every cancer cells are similar. For case, colon cancer plus breast cancer cells repeatedly have diverse gene modification that assist them produce or extend. Even amongst different group by means of colon cancer, the disease can have diverse gene modification.

But now as cancer cells can have a lot of diverse gene modification, these tablets can attack lots of unusual targets. These influences may be supportive against, and which side affects every drug can be the basis.

Some under attack drugs are additional "targeted" than others. A number of may target solely odd protein in cancer cells, as others can have an effect on quite a few diverse proteins in cancer cells. Others presently boost the method that is the body brawl the cancer cells. Once more, this can have an effect on wherever these drugs put in addition to what side effects they cause.

Targeted drugs are frequently collected by how they effort or what fraction of the cubicle they bother.

Many different types of targeted therapies are used to treat cancer, and many more are being developed.

Targeted drugs come in 2 main forms:

- Monoclonal antibody drugs are man-made versions of large immune system proteins (called *antibodies*) that are intended to hit a very precise target on cancer cubicle. These kinds of drugs are at times referred to as *biologics* since they are prepared in existing cells. The broad names for these pills (as opposed to the brand names) for case, rituximab, panitumumab, etc.

- Small-molecule pills are substance like other form of pills. They are not regarded as antibodies. As antibodies are huge molecules, these other pills are now and then called *small-molecule* besieged drugs. The broad names for the majority of these pills end in for exemplar, imatinib, dasatinib, etc. Besieged medicines can be a cluster by how they function or what portion of a unit they target. A small number of widespread types of besieged therapies are scheduled here, although this is not an inclusive. Many diverse besieged medicines are being exploited, and new medicines are coming out all the time.

Signal transduction inhibitors

The cubicle in the bodies usually produces or stops increasing in reply to substance signals they select from the region around them. These indicators are spread during proteins to the cubicle's control hub which tells what to act. In cancer units, these signals from time to time get wedged in the "on" place, telling the unit to develop even devoid of getting an exterior signal.

Some besieged medicines obstruct proteins that are sign for cancer cubicles to nurture. Jamming these cell indicators sometimes assist in keeping the cancer in control, even though it's not obvious if some of these pills alone can heal cancers. Few of these pills are exploited by themselves, as others are exercised along with further cure, for exemplar chemo.

Immunotherapy is healing that utilizes your body's own resistant system to aid in fighting cancer. Obtain details about the diverse kinds of immunotherapy in addition to the sort of cancer utilized to take care of.

What role does immune system perform?

Your immune organism is a compilation of organs, individual cells, and material that help defend you from illness and a number of ailments. Immune cells furthermore the substances they build trek all the way to defend it from microorganisms that cause illness. They also assist in guarding you from the disease in some manner.

It may help to think of your body as a castle. Germs like viruses, bacteria, and parasites are like hostile, foreign armies that are not normally found in your body. They try to invade your body to use its resources, and they can hurt you in the process. Your immune system is your body's defense force. It helps keep invading germs out, or kills them if they do get into your body.

The immune system keeps track of all of the substances normally found in the body. Any new material in the human body that the resistant system doesn't know raises a panic, causing the unaffected system to hit it. Substances that is the reason an immune reply are known *antigens*. The resistant response can wipe out anything having the antigen, like germs otherwise cancer cells.

Germs have stuff on their exterior surfaces, like particular proteins, which are not in general set up in the body. This immune organism sees this distant material as antigens and hit them.

Cancer cubicles are also diverse from standard cells in the human body. They now and then have odd stuff on their external surfaces that can be active as antigens. However germs are awfully different from usual human cubicle and are repeatedly easily seen as distant, but cancer cells and standard cells have smaller amount of clear disparity. On account of this, the resistant system doesn't for all time know cancer cells as strange. Cancer cells are fewer similar to soldiers of an assaulting army and more similar to traitors inside the lines of the human cubicle populace.

Kind of cancer immunotherapy

Numerous types of cancer healing can be considered of as immunotherapy.

A number of rouse your own resistant system to clash the illness. This can be through either by increasing the immune method in a very wide-ranging way, or by guidance the immune structure to hit some component of cancer cells purposely.

Other treatments now and then thought of because immunotherapy employ immune system parts that are prepared in the laboratory. A small number of them augment the immune collection previously whilst in the body. Others don't in fact have an effect on the resistant system. In its place, the antibodies themselves aim definite proteins that assist cancer cells nurture. Through fastening toward these proteins, these antibodies end cancer cells from mounting or make them expire. These kinds of antibodies are as well identified as *targeted remedy*.

The major sort of immunotherapy now being exercised to treat cancer is discussed here. They comprise:

Monoclonal antibodies: These antibodies are artificial explanation of resistant method proteins. Antibodies could be extremely helpful in curing cancer since they can be intended to assail a very exact portion of a cancer unit.

- Cancer vaccines: Vaccines are stuff insert into the human body to create an immune retort against definite diseases. We generally reflect of them when being specified to healthy natives to help put off illness. But a number of vaccines can assist stop or heal cancer.
- Unclear immunotherapy: These treatments improve the immune coordination in a wide-ranging mode, nevertheless this can yet aid the immune system assails cancer cells.

Immunotherapy medicines are now utilized to treat lots of diverse kind of cancer.

Hyperthermia to cure Cancer

Hyperthermia is a body heat that is high than usual. High body heat is often occurs by illnesses, like fever or heat up hit. However hyperthermia can also relates to heat healing – the cautiously limited employ of heat for checkup use. Here, we will center on how warmth is exercised to cure cancer.

While cells in the human body are out in the open toward higher than standard temperatures, transformation occurs in the cells. Warmer temperature can make the units more possibly to be affected through other healing such as rays therapy orchemotherapy. Exceptionally high heat can eradicate cancer cells complete, but they as well can harm or kill standard cells plus tissues. This is the reason hyperthermia have to be cautiously controlled and ought to be completed via doctors who are skilled in utilizing it.

The proposal of using high temperature to heal cancer has been approximately for some time; nevertheless untimely attempts had diverse results. For case, it was tough to continue the accurate temperature in the precise area while restraining the things on other components.

But at the moment newer tools lets better control as well as more exact release of warmth, and hyperthermia is exercised against numerous kinds of cancer.

There are 2 diverse paths in which hyperthermia possibly be exercised:

Extremely high temperatures are employed to wipe out a minute spot of cubicles, like tumor. This is repeatedly known as *hyperthermia* or else *thermal ablation*.

The heat of a component of the body could be elevating a few degrees upper than usual. It aids other cancer cures like emission, immunotherapy, or chemotherapy functions better. This is known as *regional hyperthermia* or complete-*body hyperthermia*.

Local hyperthermia utilizes very lofty heat

Local hyperthermia is employed to warm up a minute area such as a tumor. Extremely high heat is used to destroy the cancer units through coagulating the proteins inside them and demolishing close by blood vessels. As a consequence, this cooks the region that is uncovered to the warmth. Radio effect, microwaves, ultrasound effect, and other type of power can be utilized to warm the region. While ultrasound is exercised, the method is described as *elevated amount focused ultrasound*

The warm may be useful in different techniques:

- **Exterior:** High energy effects are expected at a tumor close to the body facade from a mechanism outer side of the human body.
- **Internal:** A slim needle or explore is inserted into the tumor. The tilt of the search releases power, which warms the tissue about it.

This Radiofrequency ablation is most likely the most universally used sort of limited hyperthermia. It employs high-energy radio effect for healing. A thin, needle-like search is inserted into the tumor designed for a short instance, usually 10-30 minutes time frame. Placement of the search is guided via ultrasound, MRI, or else CT examination. The tilt of the explore places out a high-frequency existing that generate warm (between 122° plus about 212°F) as well as wipe out the cells inside a definite area. The lifeless cells are not distant, but turn into scar tissue plus reduce in size as time passes.

RFA is most frequently used to heal tumors that is difficult to be detached with operation or meant for patients who are unable to go during the stresses of surgical treatment. It can frequently be completed while an outpatient. RFA might be recurring for tumors that approach or start to develop. It can too be included to other cure like surgery, emission therapy, chemotherapy, hepatic arterial mixture therapy, alcohol ablation, or else chemoembolization.

RFA is employed to cure tumors up to around 2 inches crosswise. It is nearly all commonly employed to cure tumors inside the liver, kidneys as well lungs, and is considered for employ in other region of the body. Lasting outcomes after RFA healing are not so far known, but premature fallout are hopeful.

The cancer cure alternatives that your doctor suggests depend on the kind and phase of cancer, potential side effects, as well as the patient's choices and generally health. In cancer heed, different sorts of doctors frequently function together to develop a patient's overall cure strategy that unite different kinds of healings. This is known as multidisciplinary. Cancer inconsistency arises when there are dissimilarity in the occurrence, rate, death, and load of cancer that be present among particular population groups, including racial and cultural minority assemblage.